M000190725

Resilience Rising

Stories of Miscarriage, Infant Loss, Infertility and Finding Joy After Pain

Visionary Authors:

Dr. Shantell Chambliss

Courtney Shorter

Co-Authored By:

Ngozi Baker

Dr. Donnisha B. Davis

Michele Minor

Tiffany Thompson

Terika Williams

Preface by Ngozi Baker

Printed in the United States of America.

ISBN: 978-1-7347994-1-5
Edited by Joi Donaldson

TABLE OF CONTENTS

PREFACE

By Ngozi Baker

The journey to write this book has been many years in the making for each writer. Many of us have shied away from sharing our stories in written word from fear that it will be scrutinized, misconstrued, and remain in print long after we've passed on to glory. We've sown a myriad of emotions (i.e. joy, excitement, sadness, nervousness, anxiety) into this project and are prayerfully hoping it helps at least one person who’s gone through or is considering this journey to feel seen and understood... We are Resilience Rising!

Lily in the Valley:
Pressing Towards Joy & Freedom

by Ngozi Baker

I dedicate this chapter to God, my loving husband and our beloved son! I appreciate each of you always ranking highest as my greatest cheerleaders.

Our anthology offers various families' perspectives. My own will provide a bird's eye view of what is not commonly spoken about - health challenges, divine interruptions for a future God-appointed time, as well as the highs and lows of marriage that may occur as a result of one's infertility journey and a budding mother-child relationship once the miracle child is born.

Our Love & Summation: The Infertility Journey

My husband and I are an eHarmony success story which I'm very proud to tell anyone! God can bring people together in all kinds of ways and the internet is one! We quickly bonded as we shared our stories of the past, the good and bad, our desires for the future, and all the possibilities that could occur through sharing a life together. We married two years later in the fall of 2011 surrounded by some of our closest family and friends.

Our infertility journey summarized in five sentences - One for the books! Journey of a lifetime! A *FAITH* walk like no other! You never know who you're raising! Resilience rising!

The beginning of our fertility journey was quite unique for me. Initially, I learned of my own upon graduating from undergrad when I was diagnosed as a woman who'd developed PolyCystic Ovarian Syndrome (PCOS). I was filled with mixed emotions from gratitude that I finally knew a name for what I was experiencing to sadness not knowing what lied ahead in my future. I was also in shock feeling my body had failed me, wondering how one could experience being fertile for several years then almost feeling with a finger snap of a couple of years later it was gone. Unfortunately, by the time we married and were ready to begin growing our family two years later, we'd learned through the years we'd developed three infertility factors between us. In addition to PCOS, I learned I'd developed another infertility factor, a microadenoma (a very small noncancerous tumor on my pituitary gland) requiring medication to inhibit lactation production when not pregnant. What's crazy is I began noticing what I thought was nipple discharge years prior only to then learn I'd been lactating while *not* pregnant! I presumed I'd done my due diligence in consulting with a medical professional regarding the "discharge," but they passed it off as not a big deal after additional breast evaluations; thus, I never consulted an

Endocrinologist for further evaluation. After receiving this information we knew we'd require the help of a Reproductive Endocrinologist to achieve the dream of carrying our own child(ren). If only it were that simple! During our initial consultation we met the Reproductive Endocrinologist, Fertility Nurse Coordinator and the clinic's Financial Counselor. We learned about the basics of the available fertility treatment options and what would be our best and only option, In Vitro Fertilization (IVF) given our infertility factors and my complex medical history.

We were also informed that I'd be required to lose 20 pounds before qualifying to begin our treatment regimen as well as the shocking cost. We walked out of the office that day a little disappointed from all we'd just learned as it felt so unattainable in that moment. I can vividly recall feeling devastated after several additional months of praying and our inability to become pregnant miraculously on our own. I felt defeated even fasting and being diligent in seeking God's face because there was still no baby. I wanted so badly for my God to "show" our Reproductive Endocrinologist His power by us being one of those couples who were once told they couldn't do it on their own and then it miraculously occurring. However, over time I realized my motivation in the need to say, "See, told ya my God was greater!" was completely wrong and humbled myself going back to the fertility clinic months later for a secondary consultation. Little did I know, God would show *me* He was greater. However, it wasn't about proving His power to someone else nor how our child's conception would occur as the miracles He possessed, but that the power to perform would be by *His will* and in *His divine timing*!

Given the anticipated cost, we became open to considering other options of fulfilling our dream of parenthood through the help of a gestational carrier or adoption. Oddly, IVF was the least expensive of the options so we began the process. Unfortunately, by the time we were finally ready to begin our IVF treatment, the cost had increased due to the new coverage year. As a result, we opted on taking out a second mortgage on our home as to not deplete our savings. Fortunately, my insurance carrier at the time was Aetna which was the only federal employees' health benefits plan offering the highest coverage (50%) of the fertility treatment cost. Sadly, the days of this type of coverage for us federal employees came to an end by the next open enrollment season. I never understood why this decision was made as it appears more women and men face infertility factors than ever before. I did inquire in writing of both Aetna and OPM as to their decision to discontinue this coverage, not solely for my benefit but for those who needed this necessary support. I was told during the years that the federal employees' health benefits plan offered a robust fertility package many often dropped shortly after no longer needing their services.

Our fertility process did not go as "planned" with so many factors being completely out of our control. It was not fluid and we encountered many bumps along the way. Some examples were me becoming seriously ill requiring hospitalization for a week after a beach vacation with my husband. Unfortunately, at discharge the extent of my diagnoses was unknown. I immediately followed up with the recommended Otolaryngologist (aka ENT) where they were able to quickly connect the dots, diagnosing me by placing a videostroboscopy through my nostril down to my larynx. We learned the secondhand smoke I inhaled while having a romantic evening walk past one of the boardwalk restaurant's patio precipitated not only my asthma attack but also caused me to develop an irritable larynx, Laryngopharyngeal reflux (LERD), and a vocal cord paralysis. You're likely wondering how this correlates to my IVF process. Well, this illness and hospitalization occurred within less than 10 days before we were scheduled to begin our 2016 IVF journey. Unfortunately, we were told we'd have to delay our cycle to allow my body to fully heal. I was extremely frustrated because by this time it had taken so much for me to even consider going through with the treatment due to some of the potential health complications and just when I was ready to plunge forward, it was ripped away!

Ten months later, we were back on pace for our IVF journey to begin. We'd gone through several hours of necessary appointments (i.e. attending medication administration courses, therapy including support group and individual sessions, various medical appointments and diagnostic measures including genetic counseling with the Maternal Fetal Medicine (MFM) specialist due to my complex medical history, etc.). I'd learned to trust my husband on a deeper level by having faith in him to administer the intramuscular fertility medication while administering my own subcutaneous fertility and anticoagulant medications. We spent hours in prayer seeking God's wisdom in whether my illnesses meant we'd never conceive and carry our own child. By this time, I'd worked my butt off to accomplish the goal of losing nearly 40 pounds to qualify as a fertility candidate by following the "My Healthy Plate" model, increasing my water intake and light physical activity (mostly walking) when motivated.

Our IVF journey towards "Baby Baker" officially kicked off on April 22, 2016 which is a special date that's near and dear to our hearts. When initially sharing our anticipated start date and soliciting prayers some loved ones assumed we'd selected the date knowing the significance but it was ALL in God's perfect plans and His timing! The date had actually been selected by our fertility clinic based on my last several menstrual cycles and like clockwork it came just as anticipated (which is rare for women who live with PCOS)! The ball literally began rolling at a very quick pace thereafter and it seemed we'd only had time to focus on strictly adhering to our treatment plan (i.e. follow-up monitoring appointments (almost daily and literally at the crack of dawn as it was still dark when leaving the house. Ugh!), being poked and prodded checking my follicle counts, hormone levels); working; and being as intentional as possible in purposefully taking time for ourselves and one another. Although it may be read with ease, it wasn't easy to go through during this time. There were many days of mixed and singular emotions like frustration, anxiety, disappointment, joy, and excitement.

Our egg retrieval day was Wednesday, May 4th, which was determined by the size of my follicles. Once the follicles reached their optimal size, another reproductive endocrinologist from my fertility clinic performed the egg retrieval. The procedure was performed under anesthesia in their operating room by removing all of my available eggs from within each follicle where the eggs were housed. They conducted this procedure by aspirating as many eggs as possible with a needle being repeatedly inserted into my ovaries (where the follicles are located). I'm sure someone's reading this in horror but I promise it sounds a lot longer than it actually took and for the most part is usually minimally painful. The procedure took approximately 15-20 minutes minus the additional time in the recovery room. I was released when I was well enough to go home to rest.

Although we knew going in that no two IVF cycles were alike (as treatment protocols differ depending on one's health history and the cause of their infertility), we were not ready for what happened when I was placed on bedrest the next day. In general, women's ovaries in their natural state are the size of a grape. However, my body responded exceptionally well to my regimen that I ended up with more than the average follicle count in my ovaries for a typical IVF cycle. By the next day, my ovaries measured the size of an orange! Although some may believe it was good news, it left me in a lot of pain. Not from the retrieval procedure itself but from how enlarged my ovaries had become. They bore down on nearby organs until they decreased to their normal size. For those who've been through fertility treatments, you're familiar with Ovarian Hyperstimulation Syndrome (OHSS) and what it likely meant moving forward. For those unfamiliar, the fertility treatment overstimulated my ovaries, causing them to produce more eggs than usual (typically one egg per menstrual cycle).

The great news was they'd RETRIEVED 13 EGGS from my ovaries which was OUTSTANDING! I had four times the desired amount for a single IVF cycle! Once my eggs were retrieved, the embryologist immediately attempted to fertilize each one with a single sperm from my husband's sample collected earlier that day. Next, our fertilized eggs were placed in an incubator to grow into embryos. By the next day, 6 of the 13 embryos continued to grow. Over the next five days, we were provided with updates on their progress. Unfortunately, as the days passed, we continued to learn of more being lost resulting in us being left with only three embryos. We knew some could be lost but until it happened, I didn't know how much I loved every single embryo. Simply loved because they were a by-product of us made through God's help in modern science!

This is where our process may differ from the "average" IVF cycle. We elected to pay for an additional step in which DNA was biopsied from each embryo for testing. As we'd researched the process of IVF, we learned of the advances in technology through the years where this test could be used as a predictor of potential miscarriages once the embryo was transferred into the mother's uterus. This test could also be used to help medical professionals and parents be aware of genetic factors throughout the pregnancy and birth which could play different roles throughout the child's life. We also pre-planned an elected brief pause in our cycle to freeze our remaining embryos for 2-4 weeks while we awaited the genetic testing results and during that time take additional fertility medication to prepare my uterus for our *single* Frozen Embryo Transfer (FET).

However, in similar theme, our plans did not occur as mapped out prior to starting our journey. Remember me mentioning overstimulating a moment ago? Well, that threw in a monkey wrench although we knew it could've been a possibility. You see, in our mind, we'd have our FET in July and within a few weeks, we'd know whether we were expecting a new family member over the next several months. We thought the hardest part was over and were both excited about the possibility of parenthood starting before we knew it. But due to overstimulation, our wait pushed up four months, allowing my body to heal for an optimal FET and a prayerful anticipated pregnancy. By this point, we'd lost another embryo with only two remaining. I began slipping into depression after the genetic test results revealed one of our babies test was inconclusive and the other had Trisomy 22. Our fertility clinic informed us of our options which was to either thaw and retest the embryo whose results were inconclusive (think thawing meat then refreezing and the potential unfavorable result when thawing again) OR leave them as-is with the hopes of a positive outcome proceeding without the additional information (as with most pregnancies). Unfortunately, we also learned from our clinic that they were not willing to proceed with an FET for our baby that had been determined to have Trisomy 22 as they only used embryos with the highest chances for survival. The pain began to feel insurmountable and my depression deepened. My husband and I prayerfully sought God to determine whether we should re-thaw our surviving embryo, understanding they too could be lost through that process or do nothing and proceed with an FET in the near future. After a few days, we reconvened, sharing what God had spoken to us individually and it was the same message: to take our chance keeping them frozen until the appointed time! This type of powerful confirmation still brings me chills!

I was determined to survive this difficult time because that's one thing I do best! I also began allowing Satan to reign freely in my thoughts, spoon-feeding me all kinds of nonsense. It was during this time that I began to withdraw from my dear husband, carrying the guilt that I couldn't have children with the man of my dreams the "normal" way. I replayed the toxic thoughts in my head that perhaps if he'd married someone else, he could achieve his dream of fatherhood. At one point, I'd even built up the nerve to have the courageously painful conversation with him that I'd understand (not 100% true) if he'd want a divorce knowing his desire for children. He lovingly told me that all couples have their "thing" and this was just ours; that we'd be okay and we're a family together with or without children. He expressed his love for me first and foremost above his desire to become a father which only deepened my love for him!

After that conversation, I was able to remember I couldn't allow the disappointment or pain (physical, emotional, psychological) I was experiencing to overtake me so I fell back on what I knew was true. I called on God while reminding myself that "I can do all things through Christ." I knew God was proud of my growth in totally relying on Him. I literally had to keep telling myself throughout the day, "I got this!" and "You [both me and God] can get through this!" Yes, I'm a Christian woman but if I'm completely honest, I also cursed Eve at least once for giving into temptation of the forbidden fruit and the turmoil for women that ensued thereafter. So happy no matter what I've gone through, God always manages to allow for my sense of humor to remain intact! However, in all seriousness, this was a process and it took a couple of months to reach this point.

The Toll and Joy in the Making

Our fertility journey took an emotional, mental and physical toll on not only my husband and me individually, but also our relationship with one another. The relationship my husband and I have worked so hard to maintain up to this point is very different from how it began 12 years ago and certainly from when we made our covenant with God before some of our dearest family and friends 10 years prior. We were NOT prepared for what we were to face during our infertility journey. Back when it started, only a few people openly shared their journeys. It was as if one carried a badge of shame believing they were considered as "defective" or even "broken" so it was kept hidden, leaving them grieving in private. I, on the other hand, tend to be more of an open book and knew I couldn't do this journey alone. I drew strength from my best friends, a select few family members, husband, therapist (definitely get you one) and God. When we began planning our family, I believe I only knew of one close friend who'd shared in a similar experience. Theirs resulted in two beautiful babies born through Intrauterine Insemination (IUI) who I'm honored to watch grow throughout the years. My husband and I have had to fight like hell even with one another to uphold our marital commitment of divorce not being an option by investing our time and energy in participating in our church's infertility and marriage ministries. We obtained marriage mentors along with individual and marital counseling. If you recall, I spoke of the weight loss journey I had to undergo in order to qualify for our IVF treatment. Unfortunately, one of the aftermaths of this journey has been regaining back all the weight lost within three years of giving birth. However, I'm finally learning to love and accept the skin I'm in while progressing towards a healthier lifestyle.

I have three very special memories of my fertility journey. Our journey was very planned with many aspects we had absolutely no control of so, to an extent, certain memories are permanently ingrained within my psyche with some I'm happy to have which elates me. I can still vividly recall the day my husband and I went to the fertility clinic for our pregnancy test after our frozen embryo transfer. I was five weeks pregnant and had a strong inkling the morning of because that day I'd been urinating more than usual. I mentioned it to my husband as we drove home from the fertility clinic. I shared I thought we were pregnant but he was a little skeptical. He shared his apprehension with wanting to believe we were expecting, desiring to reserve his joy for confirmation to avoid disappointment, which I understood and respected. Once home, we prepared to go our separate ways for work. However, I knew I was going to get that confirmation call later that afternoon. Sure enough, later that afternoon we learned that we were pregnant. I immediately called him at work to share the news which he was so happy to receive. I believed I may have even cried tears of joy at our dream coming to fruition.

Key takeaway: Trust your body and intuition as it wouldn't be the first nor last time it served me well. My second very special memory was the first time I felt the butterfly flutter of my "little" (the name I affectionately call little ones) moving around within me. Some may describe it as gas, which it eventually felt like once he grew much larger, but those initial times felt like a light-feathery touch on the inside of me to say, "Hi mommy, I'm really here!" My third favorite memory was laying on the bed talking to my husband at 26 weeks gestation dreaming of our future with our dear son-shine. Our son started kicking and my husband had never experienced feeling a baby's kick. He gently laid on my tummy and I began tearing up while singing, "Jesus loves me this I know, for the Bible tells me so…" My husband not only heard his son but also felt his touch reacting to him being near. Within moments, he also felt our son-shine moving along his face. It was pure joy and happiness which we captured it in a photo to cherish forever. When I am able to step outside of myself, especially on those really tough days, these memories give me the reassurance that God IS real!

Our pregnancy, as with our fertility journey, was filled with many ups and downs due to health challenges for both our son and me. Three of the most unexpected occurrences were 1. Learning the pain I'd been experiencing in my legs waking me in the middle of the night was Post Thrombotic Syndrome resulting from the multiple deep vein thrombi in my calves from four years prior. 2. Our son stopped growing at 34 weeks gestation resulting from being intrauterine growth restricted (IUGR) and remained classified as Small for Gestational Age (SGA) which he'd remained until born 19 days later at 4 pounds, and 3. Our son being admitted to the Neonatal Intensive Care Unit (NICU) at five hours old due to having my husband's blood type which was not compatible with my own once we were detached from one another. Understandably, after all I'd been through over the past few years up until that point within less than 6 weeks of birthing our son-shine, I was on edge and a nervous wreck. I immediately sought help from a local mental health crisis center at the recommendation of my OB-Gyn after receiving an emergency call from my very concerned husband. It was then when I was diagnosed as a person who suffers from Post-Traumatic Stress Disorder (PTSD), Postpartum Anxiety, and Postpartum Depression and I continue to live with the effects of these disorders to this day. Sadly, living with these diagnoses challenged my ability to foster the desired relationship with our son. However by now you've learned I'm no quitter - I'm a fighter! Our story doesn't end there!

I thought I'd never be able to physically carry my own child(ren). Yet, here we are today and our son-shine is a walking testimony and miracle! I was able to carry him until birth, despite the challenges we faced together, which has been an expression of our resilience. I'm in awe of all God has brought me through, even as a woman who's experienced infertility.

I was prompted to share my story as I'm a Black woman in America with the Maternal-Child health crisis happening within our community. I recall desperately praying, openly talking to my husband, OB-Gyn and MFM about my desire for both me and our baby to survive the pregnancy and delivery. I remember, while carrying our son, learning of Kira Johnson's tragic birth story shortly after delivering her 2nd son. It devastated me to learn she was no longer alive to enjoy her husband and their 2 beautiful sons because no one listened to their concerns. Kira's story terrified me. To think I too could become a statistic and be unable to enjoy the beautiful life I desired with my husband and son. I'm grateful for the great obstetrics team who listened when I openly shared my desire of wanting to live and enjoy our lives together. My concerns were understood and validated by my OB-Gyn, her being willing to advocate for us to my MFM when she thought it would be best to deliver rather than risk potential negative ramifications by allowing our son to remain in utero any longer.

Kira's story also inspired me to fiercely advocate for Black mamas and the future generations we carry!

My current life is very different than before but continuing to have my tribe (You know who you are!) has helped me tremendously. I have different people serving in the various categories of my life, as I do in theirs. I've learned to prayerfully and lovingly open up even more to my husband and vice versa. Our relationship has faced some serious challenges since before starting our fertility journey and Satan desperately desires victory. Unfortunately for him, we fight back harder! We've been challenged to overcome the intrusive thoughts of dishonoring our covenant and considering whether to opt for divorce. Our most desperately sought after love-child and new whirlwind life together had us questioning it all. These thoughts were the most painful to endure. Fortunately, we recognized them as just another trick of the adversary. We recognized he desired our seed [son] and the surest way to him was to steal, kill, and destroy our union.

Today's overall feel in our relationship is: we're making it! Doing our best to not only continue to survive but THRIVE daily! We've learned how to thrive through our individual and marital relationships with God, individual and couples counseling, the life application of various books we've read and conversing with married couples and parents about the meaning of "doing whatever it takes," for daily success in our marital and parental-child relationships.

I'd say I'm currently "somewhat" living a reimagined life as none of this has been what I desired many years ago! Nonetheless, I've begun to intentionally experience moments of joy rather than simply allowing life to unfold.

The dark clouds that've been looming over our nuclear family's heads for so long are starting to drift, allowing more sunlight to brightly shine.

Even my maternal-child relationship with my son is in a new season. We experience one another through intentionally curating fun atmospheres which makes room for laughter, joy, peace and calmer conversations. We love one another so tenderly and encourage each other effortlessly. He's my little buddy and I'm so proud to have been hand-picked as his mommy.

I am now committed to regaining joy daily! Things I've individually done to help foster this commitment into my life/our lives has been re-engaging in my love for audiobooks (cause let's face it, I'm a busy mama and wife who rarely has moments to sit down and delve into a book) on various subject matters (i.e., Relationships (with God, marriage, parenting, friendships), and autobiographies of interest). I've also learned the value of pouring more into myself through well spent alone time including weekends hotel getaways enabling me to do things how and when I want because I was a *whole* person before becoming a wife and mother. I intentionally induce laughter, dine, watch TV, movies, and documentaries alone, try new recipes or cook more of my favorites. I've reaffirmed sowing into some of my passions (i.e. Women's, Maternal & Child Health Disparities, Racial Inequities in Healthcare, Healthcare Delivery and Disparities Research, and Pain Management). Simply reprogramming my brain to recall I too am just as important as anyone else I pour into has done wonders! THERAPY!!! It is the best hour to 90 minutes I spend on myself weekly tackling various subjects (i.e., grappling with who I am and not what's happened to me, our marriage, parenting, and acquiring trauma survival skills related to the death of my parents (mother 11 years ago and my father 6 months ago), previous employment experiences, and exhausting unfavorable encounters with the US healthcare system (my own and various family and friends, etc.). It's the closest thing to consistent self-care on an ongoing basis I experience. Lastly, intentionally fostering deeper relationships with God, my husband, our son, our family and friends helps to bring me closer to complete healing.

I can't say I'm completely healed from all aspects of my fertility journey and its aftermath but I'm in the healing process. Something I still grapple with is whether my desire to mother a second child will ever be fulfilled in this lifetime. We've made the decision to not carry another child due to the challenges we faced not only with my life but also our son's while pregnant. I've prayed for the desire to be removed for years yet, at least 3 years later, the yearning hasn't disappeared. I do accept that this child may not come from my flesh but there's always room for the miraculous blessing of adoption (we don't have the $30K+ needed to make it a reality and are still paying on the loan we took out for IVF). It especially stings when asked by well-meaning people whether it's "time for another one". They have no idea the depth of internal pain I bear regarding this subject. Nonetheless, I still must find a way to cultivate joy. Joy for the life I'm able to live in spite of my past and current circumstances. Joy for the child of my flesh I can pour into now and the other children whom God has strategically placed in my life. So, I encourage you to remember: this is the day to choose life - your life - and live it joyfully!

God's joy continues to be present in my life and some days it's more apparent than others. I am often simultaneously juggling more than I should, making it difficult to experience the joys around me. Proudly, I confess to still be a work in progress (seeking God, practicing mindfulness and other health and spiritual modalities, actively participating in therapy, and taking my physical and mental health medications). Being a work in progress means I'm able to wave my hands through the clouds (my many challenges) breathing in new life. Our infertility journey has been well worth it today, most of all for being able to experience our 5-year-old son (going on 80, my "Old Man Sam" as I affectionately call him). He's such a light and a character! I don't know what God has in store for his path but I truly know it's great and I pray we live a long life experiencing it alongside him! He's our "Lone Survivor" (also affectionately called) of all his siblings and a mighty warrior. He's highly intelligent, strong-willed, tenacious and possesses more grit than many I know, leaving some to question whether he's only 5 years old. However, anyone who's ever encountered him or heard his story can attest no truer words have been spoken of him.

I share my experience as I know I didn't live through it just for me. This experience is for others as well. Choose to boldly live out God's purpose in your life daily; not perfectly, but imperfectly perfect! I've now lived long enough to know life gets messy the longer you live it (no happily ever after here) with many peaks and valleys. However, the great question is "what are you going to do when life doesn't occur as desired? Marvel at it? Endlessly sulk? Be stuck surrendering in defeat? Choosing to not thrive? Or will you find your way to enjoy it in spite of what you've been through and still desire. In truth, I constantly remind myself that I have one life to live and ponder about my legacy. I remind myself that my life is meaningful, whether I'm given everything desired or not! I choose to make life happen joyfully in spite of circumstances. Trust, I don't always reside here; some days are doom and gloom (more frequently than I'd care to admit). Nevertheless, I try to get up daily remembering as I heard many Sunday morning church services begin, "This is the day that the Lord has made, I will rejoice and be glad in it!" We've been on a journey to get here and it's been worth every ounce of pain and tears sown over the past 9 years. I've learned we can't reap without sowing, as sowing helps to bring a bountiful harvest blessing. As I prepare to enter into my 40th year of life, I'm living out the themes of being fearless, searching inward and leaning into being present with a "now or never" attitude. I continue to seek the answers to the "what ifs?!" in life and am destined to reclaim my joy.

Ngozi Baker is a Registered Nurse (17 years) and Lay Christian Counselor (10 years) with a heart for marriage and families. She desires to passionately serve in tackling the Black Maternal-Child Health and Healthcare Disparities crises in the United States. Driven to make a difference as a medical and healthcare advocate who's a multi-trauma survivor herself, Ngozi seeks to encourage and empower others to authentically own their past and seek professional or lay help for healing to live their best lives. She delves deep when exploring her infertility journey filled with candor and a sprinkle of her natural wit. Ngozi is determined to authentically live her best life and as a recovering perfectionist, she's focusing on progress over perfection. Ngozi shares how she discovers the beauty from her ashes while sojourning through one of the darkest valleys of her life. As an overcomer by faith, she'll inspire you to resiliently rise, one paragraph at a time.

Chasing Rainbows

by Dr. Shantell Chambliss

On June 13, 2016, I gave birth to the most beautiful baby boy I've ever laid my eyes on. My husband Jesse and I named him Jayden (meaning "God has heard") James (after my father whom I lost to cancer in 2015). We had been planning, praying and waiting for Jayden for the better half of ten years. Before even meeting Jesse, I struggled with the horrible symptoms of Polycystic Ovary Syndrome (PCOS) for most of my teenage and young adult years. In those 10 years, I saw every fertility specialist, holistic healer and baby expert within a 100-mile radius of our home. I came up with plans to lose weight, cure my fertility issues and get my house (physical, mental, financial and spiritual) in order to have a baby. Every single time I started a “baby making regimen”, I slacked off and eventually abandoned ship out of sheer frustration.

In early 2015, I resolved that THIS was the year that I would fight the infertility monster and that I wouldn’t stop until I was barefoot, pregnant and eating pickles and ice cream for breakfast! I hired a personal trainer, made (another) appointment with the top reproductive endocrinologist in my area and began eating clean. By July, nothing (and I mean nothing) had happened. My fertility issues hadn’t subsided and I wasn’t any closer to being pregnant. Finally, my reproductive endocrinologist suggested what I had been trying so hard to avoid: in-vitro fertilization.

For two months we mulled it over, tried to figure out how we would come up with the 5-figure price tag, read our insurance policies backwards and forward and finally agreed that it was time.

We claimed October as our start date and it was on and popping (do people still say that???). Our first in-vitro appointment consisted of a baseline ultrasound of my uterus. That ultrasound revealed several uterine polyps that basically shut down our in-vitro plans for the time being.

Fast forward to December. I had surgery to remove the polyps and after 3 weeks of recovery the in-vitro plans were back on. *woot woot*

Fast forward again to late February. After WEEKS of hormone pills, injections, suppositories (TMI, I know), egg harvesting, sperm testing, embryo transfers, and bed rest, you guessed it, WE GOT PREGNANT!!! I couldn't believe it. I had done it! I hadn't given up! I conquered the infertility monster! *happy dance*

I immediately went into mommy mode: planning, nurturing, growing and glowing. 5 months in and I was officially a professional mommy. Nursery plans were underway, baby shower date set and shopping for little Jayden was becoming a daily event. Everything was perfect, until my cervix opened 19 weeks too early.

I was having one final girls night out before the baby arrived. As I chair-danced to Beyoncé's "Formation", I was in the beginning stages of labor. After the concert and back at my hotel, I began to feel a weird pressure below my navel. I couldn't get comfortable. By 4am, my best friend noticed that I was still awake and increasingly uncomfortable. We decided to pack it up and head home to my delivery hospital. When we arrived, we didn't know what to expect. My husband met us at the ER. We were sure they were going to "sew me up" and we'd head home to continue waiting for Jayden's arrival in November. The first doctor to examine me broke the news as best she could: I was 4cm dilated and she doubted they could stop labor at this point. With Jayden coming before 24 weeks, the chance of him surviving was less than 10%.

You could literally hear our hearts break.

This couldn't be right. I was healthy. All of Jayden's ultrasounds and genetic testing had been perfect. What in the hell was going on here?

Shortly after leaving us to process, the doctor returned to share that a high risk specialist from another hospital was visiting and she thought we should get a second opinion. We agreed wholeheartedly. Dr. R came in and examined me. He agreed that I had progressed quite far but thought that a cerclage (a cervical stitch) could be a possibility if I showed no signs of infection. It would be risky and could possibly induce labor, but we were willing to try anything to turn this around. Dr. R and Dr. G agreed that they would take the pressure off my cervix in order to slow dilation and observe me for 24 hours.

I was elated. There was no way that I had an infection. I felt fine. My blood pressure was 120/80. Jayden was still kicking and moving. We were going to get the cerclage, go home and finish planning my baby shower.

The next day, Dr. R. came back and examined me. I had dilated another centimeter and my amniotic sac had moved further down into my birth canal. He admitted he had never seen anything like this and wanted to do another ultrasound to see what was going on. When he finally got my womb on the screen the first thing we noticed was that Jayden had breached himself. The day before he was head down and doing the twist (as we called it) but now his head was where his feet should be and his feet (or at least his right foot) was going in and out of my cervix!

I couldn't believe what I was seeing. This kid was kicking the amniotic sac outside of my body! Dr. R. was in awe and Jesse and I just watched his foot going in and out as if he were doing the hokey pokey.

Dr. R advised us that placing a cerclage at this point would be extremely dangerous. With the sac in my birth canal, they would have to try and place it back in my womb without rupturing the membrane. With Jayden's foot constantly pushing the sac the other way, that would be almost impossible. Even more so, he believed an infection was present although I had no symptoms. If this were true, closing my cervix could be deadly. Off the record, he told us that if I were his wife, he would not close my cervix because his gut told him that there was something wrong that we could not see.

Angry is an understatement. They have yet to invent the word to describe how we felt. I didn't have an infection so why couldn't we save my pregnancy? The doctor left Jesse and I alone to make the final decision on whether we would press forward with closing my cervix or allow labor to happen. The thought of sepsis, if I did in fact have an infection, scared us into a decision. We would allow labor to happen naturally and let God's will be done in our life.

About eight hours after we made that decision, the amniotic sac made its way fully into my birth canal. It was happening. A new doctor had just come on duty to assess the situation. As soon as he got my feet in the stirrups he told me that he had to break my water immediately. Why?? He could SEE infection in the sac. When he broke my water, the normally clear fluid, was bright yellow and smelled of raw sewage. If this infection had been present the entire time, why hadn't I shown any signs or felt sick?

Turns out that Jayden's game of hokey pokey hadn't been a game. He had breached himself and kicked the fluid filled sac outside of my womb which had prevented the infection from entering my blood stream.

54 total hours of non-medicated labor (not even a Tylenol), 6 hours of HARD contractions, 4 pushes, and lots of tears later Jayden James was here… and then he was gone. Just like that. Our perfectly planned miracle baby became an angel in the blink of an eye.

He was born so that I could live.

Jayden's autopsy later revealed that his final cause of death was chorioamnionitis and premature birth. We may never know how I contracted chorioamnionitis. According to one doctor, it's a modern-day chicken and egg conundrum. No one is quite sure whether women contract chorioamnionitis because they go into labor OR if you go into labor because you've contracted chorioamnionitis. What we do know is that one risk factor is pre-existing infections of the lower genital tract. One of those being bacterial vaginosis also known as BV or vaginitis.

In the years that have passed since Jayden came and left, grief has become a permanent resident in our home. We grieve for him every single day. We visit his gravesite often and every year we celebrate his birthday as a family as we have every year since his arrival. It's important that we never forget this pivotal moment in our lives.

Many people can't understand our grief. They view pregnancy loss as something that happens and you move on. For us, it literally brought our world to a complete stop. There have been days and weeks where we struggle to function because the grief is so great. Then there were the questions from family and friends about "trying again", medical bills from labor and delivery, mail from baby stores. Most days it's almost too much to bear.

The question I get most often is "how do you keep the faith?" In all honesty, I don't know. However, at Jayden's funeral the preacher told us that Jayden had an assignment on his life. Although his life was brief he completed his assignment. It was now up to us to complete ours.

The years following Jayden's death I dubbed "The Wilderness." Understand that the wilderness is the space between promise and fulfillment. It's not a fun place but it is fundamental. This is where our faith is put to the ultimate test. This is not a place to get angry but a place to rely fully on God. In the wilderness, friends will be scarce (or completely nonexistent), comfort will be unreachable and having faith will seem like an impossible feat. God tends to send us to the wilderness when he wants our attention. Give it to him with your whole heart and watch amazing things happen!

In 2020 we welcomed Jayden's little sister, our rainbow baby, Ryan. She is the most amazing thing to ever happen to us but, contrary to popular belief, a baby that comes after loss in no way replaces but they definitely repair. Ryan has healed our hearts, our marriage and our family in so many ways just by existing. She was handpicked by God to restore us after losing our sweet Jayden.

Shantell J. Chambliss, PhD is an award-winning entrepreneur, business strategist, advocate and philanthropist. As an entrepreneur, Shantell has developed an impressive business portfolio that includes ventures in healthcare, the nonprofit sector, consulting, retail and cultural arts. A true student of organizational development, Shantell has matched extensive education and training with over 18 years of experience as a coach and consultant to create methods that help businesses launch, grow and maximize their profit.

Shantell is the CEO and Principal Consultant of Nonprofitability, a boutique consulting firm that specializes in equipping nonprofits and faith-

based organizations with proven tools and practices that promote sustainability.

Always keeping community engagement and outreach at the forefront of her work, Shantell founded Dress for Success® Central Virginia, a Richmond, VA based affiliate of the international nonprofit organization that empowers women to achieve economic independence by providing a network of support, professional attire and the developmental tools to help women thrive in work and in life. Under her leadership, Dress for Success Central Virginia has served over 2500 women since 2012.

In 2016, Shantell and her husband Jesse experienced every expecting parents' worst nightmare when their son, Jayden, was born 19 weeks prematurely. After Jayden's passing the couple went on an in-depth journey of healing and restoration while trying to conceive their "rainbow" baby. In 2019, Shantell launched "This End of the Rainbow", an infertility and infant loss community for women of color in an effort to share resources, hope and help for other mothers of color that have experienced primary, secondary or unexplained infertility and those that are desperately chasing their rainbow.

Shantell received her Bachelor of Science in Business Administration from Virginia Commonwealth University, her Master of Business Administration from Strayer University, and her PhD in Organizational Management from Capella University, all with specializations in Human Resource Management and Organizational Development. She currently resides in Richmond, VA with her husband and daughter.

Made By Dzynne

by Dr. Donnisha Beverly Davis

If my journey was a work of art, I would liken it to Henry Matisse's "La Danse" (French for *The Dance)*. This work of art was seen as the turning point in his career as well as a celebration of life. The actual work of art and the artist relates to my journey. At some point in my loss, I knew I was going to be ok. After that, I was open. I stripped down my inhibitions and started to pursue all the things that would make me happy. It was a turning point. And everything that has come after that has been a celebration of me still being here. The figures in Matisse's work of art are stripped down of inhibitions, dancing naked in a circle, doing something that is making them happy or full of joy. I am there. I have joy now, but to understand how I got here, I need to share how it all started.

Fibroids! Seemed like 4 out of 10 black women I know have fibroids. We seemed to have different stories as to how we discovered we had fibroids, yet we all have the same story as to how we got rid of them. I discovered my fibroids after figuring out my cycle was death every 28 days. This was my early 20s. They grew and I couldn't take the pain, the getting up to use the bathroom all night, losing sleep from using the bathroom, and looking 5 months pregnant. My OBGyn told me the words I will never forget. He said, "Your fibroids are so big that if you got pregnant, the baby and the fibroids would fight for space in my uterus and the fibroids would win." Little did we know that even after having surgery, my uterus was still weak, causing the fibroids to "win space" over my baby. I had "the surgery". A laparoscopic myomectomy. The procedure was supposed to be in and out. But the doctor discovered I had way more fibroids than my scans showed. This caused him to do major incisions on my uterus. Do you see where I'm going here?

One day in February 2011, I had one of the best moments in my journey. I had that "where is my period?" moment. This led to a trip to CVS, a very nervous pregnancy test and a scared woman at the same time. I remember seeing the positive test and acknowledging that I was scared but excited to tell my people.

I carried the pregnancy well, I must say. But there were several times where I was at the ER because things didn't feel right. I remember it was a few weeks after I announced to Facebook and my social circle that I was pregnant. Here comes the worst time of my life. I remember feeling nauseous, light headed and sweaty. I called my OBGyn and he told me to call an ambulance. I think at some point I passed out. Not sure if it was before or after I put on my nice camel Tory Burch sandals (which I lost at the hospital).

I remember feeling more pain and looking up from the gurney at people rushing to poke and prod me. I was rushed into a room where more work was being done by so many people around my gurney. At some point, I signed papers concerning my possible death. I hated everything that was happening around me. I was in pain, my body temperature was so low, I didn't even think it was possible to be that cold. I also thought that the doctors working on me could have been the last thing I saw. I woke up strapped down and in the Intensive Care Unit (ICU). My family to this day cannot talk about what I looked like.

I experienced hell during those 11 or 14 days I was in the hospital. I don't know, I don't care to know and threw away my discharge papers. I even experienced an earthquake while in ICU! I would never forget the room shaking and then my petite nurse jumped on my bed to protect me from whatever was happening. An earthquake in Maryland was unheard of but that ordeal definitely added to the hell I was in.

After being released from ICU, I was placed on the cardiology floor because my heart was not right. My heart issues were caused by the emergency surgery, but I think it was because my heart was broken. My time spent on the cardiology floor was tough because I remember constantly vomiting all day, no sleep, pain, crying and placing a pillow on my incision, and going to the bathroom a lot. I was approached with the notion of holding my lifeless baby to take pictures. I was so sick that I couldn't really have that moment until I got better. Our baby girl, Dzynne Marie Davis, was in a freezer the entire time until I got better. They told me about funerals and cremation for her. I was recovering and I did not want to plan a funeral while getting my health better. I did eventually get to hold Dzynne with her dad. I didn’t know until years later that apparently the hospital gave my mom, sister, and brother the same option to spend time with Dzynne. A professional photographer took many pictures of us and I have those to cherish. She definitely looked like me.

What happened to me left me with physical and emotional scars. In order to save my life on August 22, 2011, the doctors performed an emergency cesarean hysterectomy. Thus giving me a physical scar that is vertical due to the type of life saving hysterectomy they did. Losing my baby, my ability to birth future babies, and almost losing my life left a big emotional scar on my heart.

I realized after my ordeal that I would need therapy. I tried one-on-one therapy and the therapist cried more than me. She did point me to a group called “Compassionate Friends” in Waldorf, MD. This was a group for parents who’ve lost a child from pregnancy to adulthood. It was at Compassionate Friends that I met the person who was significant to my journey. This person was a stranger and I don’t remember her name.

I was at the 7pm Compassionate Friends meeting where I shared my story with the group. I was nervous because I knew I wanted to share my story that day. I'd been coming to meetings for weeks, so I knew it was time. This stranger told me that going back into the workplace would be hard and that I need to find a place to go and cry or release when it becomes too much. It wasn't the person that was significant, but the message. I experienced pregnancy loss at 28 weeks in August 2011. I did not return to work until October 2011 and I was definitely not pregnant. I had several people who did not get the email of my loss (Yes, my manager sent an email to everyone in my division) asking me "how's the baby?". First few times, I was ok. After being asked repeatedly, I needed to find that place where I could go and release and get back to work. I remembered what that stranger said at my meeting. I knew that the conference room near my cubicle was never used and that is where I went to cry. I would take my pregnancy naps there.

While I've addressed important moments and people, there was a significant day of my journey. This was the day of "La Danse", the work of art by Henry Matisse that relates to my journey. This day was the turning point. It was a month after my loss and I went for a walk/run at the Sports and Learning Complex track. I felt euphoric, like everything will be ok. I would go to the track to run/walk several times a week after I was cleared by my doctor. Before I became pregnant, I lost a significant amount of weight by diet and exercise. So I was eager to get back out there and get the baby weight off me. Running helped with my grief. I ran several times a week. One day, the sky was a bit cloudy but sunny and I just kept looking up at the sky and thinking that my baby was "up there" looking over me. Such a significant day! The day that I knew joy would be possible. I stripped down my inhibitions and decided to pursue all the things that would make me happy. Being able to survive the surgeries and hospital stay gave me a second chance at life. It was time for a celebration: "La Danse."

To celebrate life while grieving seemed foreign to those around me. A friend of mine revealed years later that she thought it was odd that I was happy after such a tragic loss. But she also remembers my response and that is “I'm alive and I want to do all the things that bring me joy”.

Besides getting back to something that brings me joy, which is running, I wanted to do something I never did before and that was to take up sewing. I had no clue that sewing would bring me so much joy during my grief and for years to come. Three months after losing Dzynne, I enrolled in a sewing class at the local recreation center. It was a 6-week course. I never had a sewing machine and only used one in our home economics class in junior high school. I purchased a sewing machine, my very first sewing pattern and fabric and made a lovely dress. I enjoyed this class because it was a way to escape and be creative. I took the class one more time and found that I can learn a lot on youtube. After making so many garments, I started to share my creations on social media. This is when I created “Made By Dzynne”. I named my sewing business after my daughter. Dzynne would be proud of her mom.

Being a mom to a child that is no longer living is painful at times. Losing the ability to birth children of my own due to a partial hysterectomy was painful as well. Having a partial hysterectomy meant I still had eggs and could have a baby via a surrogate. My husband and I tried that route, but things came to a halt for circumstances beyond our control at that time. Yet, it is because of my husband that I am a mom. I have a stepson and stepdaughter. My stepson is a grown-up who came into my life at 15 years old. My stepdaughter is a teenager who lives with us. She is only 3 years older than what Dzynne would have been. Life is good!

Today, I am still pursuing the things that make me happy. I'm still in "La Danse".

Dr. Donnisha Beverly Davis is an all-around creative best known for her graphic design work. Her graphic design expertise are in government identity branding, publication design and logo design. She has over 25 years of experience as both a Senior Visual Information Specialist for the federal government and a freelance graphic designer. Her passion for the creative arts and design extends to clothing design, sewing and painting. Her freelance business, "Made By Dzynne", was named after her daughter and is where she provides clients creative art and design services.

She holds a Doctor of Management in Organizational Leadership from the University of Phoenix, Masters of Fine Art (MFA) in Design from Howard University and a Bachelor of Science in Graphic Design from Florida Agricultural and Mechanical University. Her goals are to obtain a masters degree in User Experience (UX) design before becoming the director of a design/art program at the university level.

She is a native Washingtonian, residing in Upper Marlboro, MD.

Promise Fulfilled

by Michele Minor

I dedicate this story To My Husband James, who has been by my side every step of the way, I could not have done any of this without you - I Love You; To Our beautiful daughters, who remind me daily of God's Greatness. To My mother; who introduced me to Christ and taught me how to pray; To My Midwife and Doula - "The Dream Team" they know who they are - I would not have been able to get through the pregnancy journey without you! You are the very best at what you do and I love you for it!; To Our tribe who encouraged us, cried with us, prayed for us, celebrated with us and who now join in community with us as we raise our daughters; and lastly to the many women, men and families who experience infertility, miscarriages, child loss and all those parts of the journey in between. Please know that Your journey is important, Your voice is powerful and that You are not alone! I pray that the words in this book will speak to your hearts and Bless who it is intended to Bless.

I never knew how much I wanted a child until I thought I couldn't have one.

I had finally found my person. I didn't know I was ready for Love, but when the gift comes your way, you know. He was a great guy; different from everything I had experienced before. We connected easily and both knew this was long-term. We talked about everything. Although, children were never really a discussion because it was almost an absolute! Of course it was going to happen. No need to discuss. Aren't children always a part of the plan – Husband, children, dog, house, car, job – they all kind of go together for most people. At least for me they did. 2005 was an amazing year! I was excited to be married to him and be his wife.

A few years into our marriage – year two to be exact - we realized that the couples who got married around the same time as we did were beginning to start their families. We didn't think too much of it, but it was the first time that I realized that we should probably have a discussion about having a family. As we talked about it one night over dinner, my husband shared that he wasn't ready for children right away. I definitely wanted children right away. How had we missed this? What did this mean for my career, my plans? It became a point of contention for us. Something we needed to definitely work through. What could I do but accept our current state. Pray. And Wait? Time goes on and while we were not intentionally trying, we were not intentionally trying not to become pregnant either – as marriage often goes! So, I thought maybe it would just happen. Year three, nothing. Year four, nothing. Year five our family starts to ask, "When are you all going to have some children?" They begin to act as if something was wrong with our marriage. Unbeknownst to them, we had deemed 2010 was going to be different. We had resolved that we could not control what we could not control and that we were going to take a break from the frustration and just LIVE. We celebrated our 5th anniversary and we were actually in the best place in our marriage than we had been for a while. We began to travel and really enjoy our marriage and each other. It was good, but it was definitely the calm before the storm.

Over the next year, some disappointment began to set in for me. My longing for a baby had a way of showing itself. It would show up as frustration with my husband, separation from friends, and some days, just sadness. Some days I was even quietly resentful of my husband, thinking if we had started earlier, when I wanted to, we would be in a better place by now. He is getting older, I am getting older. I could hear the elder women in the family in my head and I would tell myself, "I don't how much longer these eggs are gonna hold up! Did we miss our opportunity?" As a woman of faith, I have always been taught to be hopeful, but I was filled with so much doubt. I would pray and God would help me come back to myself, giving me a little more hope. I would then tell myself, "surely, it's coming. Right? This is only our 6th year of marriage. We still have time." Fast forward to the middle of the year and we Get A Positive! 6-10-2011 – I remember the date. So excited! All of the emotions were coming up for us. We tell our parents of course. Immediately start think of what's next. Talking daily about it. We were overjoyed that it had finally happened for us! I started eating super healthy, downloaded the pregnancy journey app, and began doing everything by the book! Anything to make sure that our baby had the best possible start. It's been about two weeks…unusual bleeding. We decide that I should go to the emergency room. I wait hours to be seen. Nervous and praying the entire time. It's my turn. After some things I don't recall, the doctor says,

“Ma’am you are no longer pregnant.”

How? How far along was I? Why do you think this happened?”

“We are unsure” was the answer to all my questions. They tried to offer solace by saying this is your body’s way of saying it just not the right time. Thanks. I had to go home to tell my husband. We shared silence and long hugs that night. Having to go back and tell our parents that we were no longer pregnant was tough. We pressed on. Vowing to keep trying. Telling ourselves, at least there is fun in the trying. You must find your joy somewhere.

We bring in the new year and as people of faith, we declared and decreed, prayed and had people pray for us. 2012 was going to be our year to have a child! We had planned a beautiful trip to Jamaica. It was finally time to go. I remember it being so peaceful and relaxing. Getting away from it all just the two of us. We had time to laugh and time to cry and just to enjoy God's beautiful landscape. I remember it being so hard to say goodbye as we headed to the airport. Home sweet home. We had been back for about four weeks and I was pretty in tune with my body at that time so I could tell pretty early that something was just not right. It was around the end of May and my normal signs were not showing up. Could this be it? I go to the store. I buy 3 different brands of pregnancy test. A Rapid, Double line, and a Yes test – I just needed to be certain. I took all of the tests and they were all negative. UUUUggghhh! A week or so passes. I am certain that something is up by now. Back to the store for 3 more tests. 3 Positives!!! We are pregnant! Again! I leave a test out in the bathroom and wait. He doesn't even notice! That is so my husband! So, I bring the test to him and share. We are both excited! This time we did things a little different. We waited to share with anyone as we were not looking forward to having another retraction conversation. This time, I found one of the best OB-Gyn practices in the area and started prenatal care as soon as possible. I drove the 40 minutes to my first appointment. The staff was friendly, always helpful when you are nervous. The Gyn came in and completed the check-up and had me do some blood work. You're 5 weeks. Very early, she says. I shared with her that we had a miscarriage the year before. She listened, gave me some follow up items and told me to take care of myself and come back in two weeks. I drove home and began to talk to my baby. "Hey baby, do you hear mommy's voice? Listen to mommy, you are going to have to fight to be here! We will get through this together." Over the next two weeks, I do all of the things you are supposed to do, took my prenatal vitamins, ate healthy, and tried to get in a little exercise. It was time to go back for my next visit. I prepare to take the 40 minute drive. As always, I pop in my favorite CD and blast my favorite Fred Hammond song: You are the Living Word. It always takes me into worship in the morning. I get there, the wait was short, we start with a regular checkup and blood work. She then requests a 7-week sonogram. It's a fairly quick visit and I head home. A couple of days later, I get a call back from the nurse. She says that my blood work came back and the Gyn wanted me to come in to discuss some things. I start thinking the worst. I tell my husband and he reminds me not to jump to conclusions and we will take it one step at a time. I make the soonest appointment that I can and take my routine 40 minute drive, overthinking all the way there. The wait is short. The Gyn comes in, asks me how I am feeling. Does she really want to know? I say I am fine but anxious to hear what she has to say. She says that my HCG levels were a little low for this stage in pregnancy and that she could not see the baby in the uterus on the sonogram. I had never heard that before. She said it was still early and sometimes the baby can be hard to locate this early. But also, it could be ectopic. What does that mean? She goes on to share that the baby is possibly in the fallopian tubes and not the uterus. Ok so, what's next? She said that we will take more blood work today and watch the HCG levels to see if they are going up. She tells me to set another appointment for a week out. I get back to the car and just start bawling. I began to pray and talk to the baby. I tell the baby to keep fighting. You belong here! I'm with you, we will get through this together. I need to get myself together because I had to go to work. I call my husband and tell him the news on the way. We pray and go on with our day. A week goes by, time for my appointment. I do my routine 40 minute drive, Fred Hammond playing and baby and I are talking. I arrive, the wait was short as usual. They request a urine sample. I wait to see the Gyn. She comes in, she performs a sonogram. She leaves the room, comes back a few minutes later. She shares that the HCG numbers have gone up and the baby is not in the uterus but actually in the fallopian tubes. She tells me again about the dangers of ectopic pregnancies and how the fallopian tube could burst as the baby grows and could cause death. She stated that we needed to act today. Does it really need to happen today? I really would like my husband to be with me. She confirmed that it needed to happen today. What does the procedure look like? She shared that they were going to give me a shot. This shot was going to reduce the baby so that it would stop growing in my tubes. What I heard was my baby was going to die today. I just talked to her this morning and told her to fight and we were in this together. This was heartbreaking. I asked the doctor for a minute by myself. I call my husband and tell him what's going on. At the end of what felt like the hardest conversation of our marriage, we know that my safety was most important. So, I move forward. The Gyn comes back in. She shares how the procedure is going to go and gives me the shot. She says that I need to come back in a week to make sure that the HCG levels continue to go down. This was the hardest ride home. I felt so sad, I couldn't even talk to the baby. I almost felt like I betrayed her. I take off of work because I just can't be around anyone. I go home and cry all day. I could not pray , I didn't want to talk, I just cried. It was the longest week ever. I take that 40 minute drive in complete silence. The wait seemed like forever. They have me take a urine sample. The Gyn comes in and asks me how I was doing. Not well. She tells me that my HCG levels have doubled since the last visit. The baby is growing. She said this is not normal. The shot usually works the first time and they need to give me a second shot. I told her that since I found out I was pregnant, I had been telling the baby to listen to her mommy and to fight to be here. She is doing just what I told her. The doctor put her hand on my shoulder and said, “you want to tell her that it's ok to stop fighting now.” I get the second shot and headed to work in silence. Later that evening, I told baby girl that I loved her and that she did her job and it was ok to stop fighting. One of the hardest things that I have ever had to do. I needed to go back in one week to test my levels again. That time they were almost at zero. The second shot worked. Just at the beginning of 10 weeks, my baby girl stopped fighting. She knew it was ok. But I was not ok. My husband and I dealt with the loss as best we could. You try to move on with normal life, but for me there was a deep sadness. This was the first time I had ever felt really depressed – without hope around being a mother. I felt like my body and God had let me down.

Healing definitely takes time. And over time I began to heal. I began to talk to God again. I asked God was this punishment for some of the mistakes that I had made in my college years? I just needed to have a reason, some understanding about why He didn't let this happen for us. You don't always get your answers fast. Sometimes the peace comes first. As I was getting better, I remember being curled up on the couch, telling God – "please don't let this be in vain. It hurts too bad. You must get Glory out of this!" In my emptiness, I told God, "You are all I have but You are all that I need." My relationship with God was changing. The type of trust that I needed to get through this was different than anything I had experienced before.

They say time heals all wounds. I definitely needed more time. I had a few things that I did to work on my healing. One of the ways was giving our baby a name. I realized that at some point I was calling her, she. I never really knew if she was a girl, but my heart knew. I prayed on her name and she will forever be remembered as Akoma – A Swahili word for love and endurance.

We took a break from the pregnancy journey. Life continued. I began to focus on my health. So many doctors said that maybe if I lost weight I could have a child. I really took that to heart. I began to take my health a lot more seriously. Losing weight became a critical focus. I did not want anything that I was in control of to prevent us from having a child. Getting the right support, eating right and exercising were working. The weight was coming down! While focusing on my health, my mother in law's health was suffering. She was diagnosed with Pancreatic cancer and it was devastating for all of us. Our focus went to supporting her and preparing for whatever this journey would bring. It was definitely on our minds that we wanted her have the opportunity to spend time with our child as things began to unfold. That, unfortunately, did not happen. She became our forever angel and went to be with our Akoma in November 2013. After this, my husband and I definitely needed something, something new, something to love. After her passing, I reached out to a church member really feeling in despair. I was probably at my most hopeless about being a mother. I shared with her how I was feeling. After listening to me, she asked me one question: “Did God say that you would have children?” I said “Yes!” I believe I heard from The Lord and the answer was yes. She gave me three words before we got of the phone: Trust In That!

Now believing our promise - we began talking a lot about options for having children. This was the first time we thought of IVF, we even discussed adoption. We had resolved not to limit ourselves. As we continued to think outside the box and our desire to care for a child increased, we began the process to become foster parents.

I knew my heart was all in - I believe my husband was only half way there, but because of his love for me, he went along with it. We began thinking through what it meant to love a child only to have them be removed from us. But we had decided that loving a child, even temporarily, was enough at this time. We began the classes, started preparing our hearts and our home. All we had to do now was wait. While waiting for a real baby. we decided to get a furbaby - Welcome Tyson! He became our love focus! I know it seems like we were looking for replacements for our grief. And that's exactly what we were doing! There were so many steps to becoming a foster parent and it was just taking so long. I began to realize more and more that my husbands' heart wasn't really in it and I am now grateful that it didn't come to fruition. It wasn't for us and it wasn't our time.

Some time passed and we made the decision to intentionally begin to try and have a baby again. While continuing my weight loss journey, I reconnected with a friend who also happened to be a midwife. We began to take walks and talk more. I shared my desire to have a baby and the challenges we were experiencing. She immediately put me on a regimen and a plan to get pregnant. While I didn't know if what she told me would work, I trusted her expertise as I didn't have any other ideas. So we did exactly what we were told. Ovulation kits, cycle monitoring, temperature checks - we did it all. Don't get me wrong, it wasn't all hard work - we had A LOT of fun too!

At this time, I really began to enjoy working out. It had become a release for me. During one of my workouts, I fell and broke my ankle. Nothing like this had ever happened to me before. This felt like yet a another hit in a series of blows. I'm in a boot for weeks and need to have surgery to repair my ankle. I prep for surgery, prior to my date and head to the hospital early the morning of September 16th, 2014. A date I will never forget. My mom and my husband were both by my side as they prepare me for the surgeon. My husband prays for me. After he prayed, strangely, the Lord told me to ask for a pregnancy test. When I asked the nurse for a pregnancy test, she told me that the surgeon was ready and that I had already told them there was no possible way I was pregnant. I could feel the irritation around my request. I persisted. They obliged. I took a test and the nurse came back and said it was positive. She said that she wanted to get me up to sonogram quickly to confirm. There on the screen I saw that perfect little dot. It was in the uterus. I was 6 weeks pregnant and getting ready to have surgery. The nurses and surgeon were so grateful that I had asked because the anesthesia could have negatively affected such a young fetus. God was looking out! Post surgery, I have a boot on my foot while going back and forth to prenatal care. This time I chose not to take that 40 minute drive but go with the person who got us here. I went back to my friend and midwife and it was the beginning of something wonderful! During one of my prenatal visits, I was diagnosed with an incompetent cervix. It was slightly open and something that we needed to watch. Due to my recent surgery, I could not work for a while and I was later placed on bedrest as the baby grew to prevent pre-term labor. The only thing I could do was rest and care for this little seed growing inside of me. God's timing is everything! Only He knew that I would need this time to nurture our baby.

After the first trimester was over, we announced to family and friends that we are pregnant! Still very nervous, but more confident than ever that this was our time. January 2015, during a church service, the Lord delivers her name: Grace! We were certainly grateful for His Grace and our Grace. The pregnancy journey had its ebbs and flows. We had an amazing community that was rooting for us, prayer warriors praying regularly and we had the best care possible.

The Final Trimester! As we prepared for Grace's arrival, my best friend, who had been by my side, planned the most amazing celebration of new life that anyone could ask for. All of the people who supported us through this time were there and we partied! Talking about it still makes me smile to this day almost 8 years later!

Time was winding down. I was determined to have a natural childbirth experience. I had prepared myself for this process mentally, physically and spiritually. I had the best midwife and doula in the area. They were supportive in making that happen. With my team and family in the room, 11 days after our 10th anniversary, Grace Laura Vivian Minor was born on May 18, 2015. We wanted her to carry power in her name so we gave her the middle name of Laura after her grandmother and my mother and Viviavn to honor James' mother. It was a beautiful birth; it took a little over an hour to deliver her naturally. It was just like I had desired. She was the absolute best gift we could have ever given to each other. We experienced unexplainable joy. This little girl brought life back into our marriage and we were going to give her the very best of ourselves.

About two years after Grace was born, we wanted to complete our family and desired to have one more child. I researched one of the best OB-Gyns in the area that dealt with women with advanced maternal age. I didn't know what to expect but knew we were ready for another child. It was at this appointment that I was told that I was "lucky" to have had Grace at my age and that based on the tests that she ran, I would not be able to have another child without some sort of "help". Although this was not what we wanted to hear, it was not devastating news for us. We began to reconcile that maybe Grace would be a singleton. Maybe God have given us all that we needed. We also knew that we could always adopt. Things were good and we were busy raising a beautifully inquisitive little girl. A couple of years passed and we had a big life change happen when Grace was about four. We needed to relocate. Move away from our family, our support system and all that we have ever known. We packed up the family, left Washington, DC and headed to our new home in

Delaware. About 6 months into our new life as we are settling in, the world turns upside down due to the Covid-19 Pandemic. Not only were we away from our community, but we were also very isolated. It was a tough time, but we were enduring. One night, I had this severe pain in my left side. We go to the emergency room. This was our first time in a hospital since the pandemic started and we were definitely afraid to be there with all of the stories that we'd heard. They took some samples to run some tests and we wait. The doctor and nurse come rushing in to the room – They say, "You Are Pregnant!" At this point, hubby and I had been told that we couldn't have children and had been through so much that we didn't even believe them. So much so, the doctors looked at our faces and asked us if we were okay. We were in shock! I shared that some years back we were told that we could not have anymore children. I told him I needed to be sure. He said we could do a sonogram. Perfect! The sonographer asked me if I knew about how far along I might be. I had absolutely no idea.

She told me that I was 8 weeks pregnant. I say, "8 weeks!? Are you serious?" She points to the screen and there she is! Unbelievable! It was Sunday, March 15, 2020 when we found out that we would become parents again! Being pregnant during the pandemic was very different. Not having our community close was challenging, but we had to press on. This little one was depending on us. I began praying for a name for her. The Lord sent me Chloe, meaning fertility or blooming. How appropriate!

I had found a wonderful Black female OB-Gyn and while my prenatal care in Delaware was good, in my heart, I knew this was not the experience that I wanted. I reached out to my dream team, my midwife and my doula from Grace's birth and they received me with open arms. We had to be creative and strategic with all that was going on. Virtual visits with my doula, prenatal yoga via zoom. I even had to temporarily move back to DC for the last part of my pregnancy to ensure that I could deliver with my midwife. We made it work! October was here and it was time for this baby to come soon. Towards the end of the pregnancy, I was diagnosed with Preeclampsia. I had never had anything like this before and it made very nervous. Because of this, I had to be induced. This was not what I planned. I thought I would have a birth similar to Grace's where I was in control, but that was far from what would actually happen. I went in for the induction on October 10, 2020. I had my heart set on Chloe being born on that day. There was something special about the date 10-10-20! I am not sure what I expected the indiction to be like, but I knew that I had the best team supporting us! Giving birth to Chloe was the absolute hardest thing that I have had to do to this date. I experienced great pain both physically and emotionally as well as a near life and death situation. I am grateful to God that my midwife and the team that He placed around me fought for me and helped us get through it. Approximately 17 hours and two epidurals later, Chloe Patricia Ann Minor was here on the day that we planned! After going through this ordeal,

I recognized that as a 45-year-old Black women, the outcome could have been very different. And for many women of color that go through this, they do not make it home. I'm so grateful to God that we made it home. After her birth, I had a lot of time to reflect. I remembered my conversation before having Grace when my friend reminded me to stand on what God had promised. He promised that we would have child(**ren**). God didn't forget even when I did. He used a plural and He meant it! Chloe being born was Promise Fulfilled. We had been fully restored!

We never expected to be parents of two children under the age of 10 at this time in our lives, but we believe that Grace and Chloe have great purpose on their lives and that our most important job is to usher them into that purpose. We have grown and matured so much since we began this journey. Now I understand that we would not be the parents that we are now if we had our children at any other time. Truly, God's timing is not our timing, but it is always right! This journey has not been easy, but it has been worth it. Through it all we stood on Jeremiah 29:11: "For I know the plans I have for you, declares the Lord, plans to prosper you and not to harm you, plans to give you a hope and a future." He has done just that and this is only the beginning.

Michele Minor was born and raised in Washington, DC and now resides in Wilmington, Delaware with her husband and two daughters. Growing up, she was a school fanatic which led to an early exposure and love for reading. If she isn't spending time reading, you can find her engaged with her favorite F's - Faith, Family, Friends and Food! She is a self-proclaimed foodie, who can break a meal down to its spices! She loves to cook for her family and considers them to be most important to her. She currently serves as a Human Resources Executive and lives by the principle of "Leaving People Better Than You Found Them." Resilience Rising is Michele's first opportunity at being an author and she is excited about where this journey will lead her.

Morgan, Ryan, and a Rainbow: Forever in Our Hearts!

by Courtney Shorter

On June 12, 2015, one day after celebrating ten years of marriage with the man of my dreams and after ten years of actively trying to have children, we experienced one of the best and most shocking days of our lives. We delivered twin daughters. They were not expected to arrive until October 2015.

I remember the day we got pregnant: January 9, 2015! We'd been going through the less invasive fertility treatments and had several failed attempts. The problem is, I have a pituitary adenoma. The best way to describe it is there's a tumor in your head that affects your reproductive system and throws all your essential hormones out of whack. In my case, the hormones that would support getting pregnant were nonexistent. Put it this way: I haven't had periods in over ten years, so the only way for me to get pregnant was with assistance. Talk about being confused and angry. Doctors didn't know or couldn't tell me why this happened to me, and the cure was brain surgery or daily medication. I opted for medication. I'd been on the highest dose for years and still no children, a period or increased hormone levels.

We finally reached out to a prominent reproductive endocrinologist in Washington DC after a traumatizing experience with one of the "chain" fertility clinics. There were millions of tests to rule out anything else and, praise God, there was nothing. The tumor was enough of a battle, but after several tries at some of the cheaper, less advanced options, there was still no pregnancy. There was Clomid, a forced period, timed intercourse. Nothing happened. Finally, the doctor recommended a procedure called forced ovulation. In my heart, I knew this would work. This was the treatment plan we needed. I was ready to go; whatever it took, I would do it. I was in the best shape of my life, mentally and physically. I lost over 150 lbs., worked out every day, and sustained a relatively healthy diet accompanied by the occasional red velvet cupcake!

Day 1. We started the nightly shots to my stomach in late November 2014 after Thanksgiving. The first one was so terrifying; to this day, I don't know if I did it right. 1 bottle of Menopure + 1 ml of the solution. Mix the solution and administer it to the belly every night. Return for bloodwork and sonogram in a week. When we returned, I was so excited. I knew my body felt different and there would be a million eggs ready to be fertilized. I was wrong. My body barely responded to the treatment. I cried. I'd done it right; why didn't it work? My doctor and nurse stayed in the room with me and explained that this was normal. Typical for who I wondered, no one else on the planet is going through this. It's only me. Of course that's not true, but having to go through fertility treatments to start your family can feel like the loneliest place ever, even though at my fertility clinic, the waiting room was FULL of people all hoping and praying for the same outcome—a child.

I returned home and increased the amount of medication for the nightly injections. By Christmas, my body was responding well, and it looked like we would be ready for the next step. Wrong again. A few more days of shots and instead of weekly bloodwork and sonograms, we are now at every other day. By January 1st, those appointments would increase to daily bloodwork and sonograms. Yes, you heard me: get up and drive 30+ minutes in hellish DC rush hour traffic every morning for a 5 min appointment. FINALLY, we are ready to make this baby. Our specific instructions were to take the ovulation injection to my stomach and then have intercourse at a particular time on a specific date. We did, and it was weird! On January 9, 2015, we had sex at 7:30 pm, and later that evening, I was getting dressed to head to my friend's birthday party at a pole dancing class. I point this out because we were given a specific window to have intercourse, and I didn't want to miss it. In my mind, missing this window also meant missing our opportunity to conceive. Weeks later, we had a positive confirmed pregnancy test. I told my best friend and my cousin. On my birthday, January 30th, I told my mom and my brother over breakfast at Busboys & Poets. At dinner later that night, I told a few other friends. It's funny that I was about six weeks pregnant by this point, and at least 30 people knew we were pregnant. We wouldn't find out until week ten that we were pregnant with twins. Much later, we found out they were both precious little girls. In contrast, only about ten people knew when we were pregnant with our son until we were 100 days away from our delivery date. We were scared to share the joy we felt as we anticipated his arrival.

While trying to get pregnant with our daughters, whom we later would name Ryan and Morgan, I realized then how taboo it was to talk about fertility issues with anyone outside of the people you felt the most comfortable with. Visiting the office, even though we were all there for the same reason, the silence in the waiting room was deafening. No one spoke to anyone except the nurses, and even then, the whisper was so low that it made me wonder if the nurse could even hear what was being said. We all know why we're in the room together, but for some reason, the fear, shame, and embarrassment of why we're here took over and everyone is quiet, not even a good morning. I mean, even in my daily life, I dreaded telling my best friend, who was also pregnant then, about what we had to do to conceive. How could she even understand, she conceived "naturally?" I use quotes here because naturally is relative, and I also know that even my sisters who've been blessed with living children, more times than not, those same sisters have experienced heartbreak in the past. My best friend asked many questions, checked in after every appointment, and made it okay for me not to be ashamed. Imagine having so many supporters in your corner but feeling so alone at the same time. That's what I felt. Not that she judged or was anything but amazingly supportive, she was the one thing that made this all okay, and to make it even better, we were now pregnant together. She was due in May and we were due in October. Our husbands were over the moon excited. She and I had already planned summer vacations and Christmas. Little did we know, we'd never have that with Ryan and Morgan.

On June 12^{th,} after a scary ambulance ride to the hospital, due to placenta abruption, we delivered beautiful our beautiful baby girls. Ryan, the big sister, was born at 1:45 pm, and Morgan, our littlest rockstar, at 1:46 pm. Born at only 23 weeks and weighing about one pound each, Ryan and Morgan looked like little red hotdogs. Although I was not allowed to see them when they were first born, I thankfully have pictures of their first few hours earthside. They were so tiny and could fit in the palm of my hands; they were smaller than the preemie diaper used to capture their first potty. Ryan and Morgan were considered micro-preemies, and babies that survive being born so early often live the first 6-12 months of their lives in a hospital Neonatal Intensive Care Unit (NICU) before going home with their families. I wish this were our story.

Life in the NICU was so hard on those little bodies. Imagine having your blood drawn every day multiple times per day, and you're not even a week old. At three weeks, Ryan had been poked more than most adults I've known. Imagine also having a blood transfusion a few times a week to replace the blood they are taking. Along with blood draws, there are daily xrays of their lungs and head. At some point in this journey, we were also notified that Ryan had a level 2 brain bleed and a virus that made it mandatory that she be separated from all the NICU babies for the duration of her stay. So, picture this: we were in the NICU and had to be in a completely separate room from everyone else. No more than one visitor at a time, gloves, gowns, hair caps, and shoe booties were mandatory. If you stepped out of the room, we had to trash our "uniform" before leaving the room, re-wash, and re-dress before we could re-enter. I remember getting dressed to go in one day, but I'd left my car key at the sink. I'd been in the room less than a minute. I had to undress at the door, trash my garments, grab my key, put it in my pocket, re-wash, re-dress, and then go back in. I'd already been there for 20 min but had only been with Ryan for 2 minutes.

To this day, seven years later, the visual of the feeding tubes, multiple IVs that moved from their arms to their feet, and the ringing bells and alarms from the incubators can still bring me to tears without warning. As parents, we sat by those incubators for hours, days, and nights at a time. NICU life is not for the weak.

When I learned we were pregnant, I felt so excited and hopeful. I felt like all the things I'd hoped for over those last ten years were finally becoming my reality. I no longer had to be just the happy "Auntie", showing up for the baby showers and birthday parties, smiling on the outside while slowly dying on the inside from guilt, grief and shame. Regret that I had to pretend to be happy for them and not sad for me. Grief that I longed for a pregnancy that had never happened and shame that my body could not do what it was "supposed to do." Finally getting pregnant, and with twins no less, we dreamed of what our girls would grow up to become. We started making plans for our lives with them in it. First words, first steps, the first day of school, a list of firsts we would never experience with them. In the blink of an eye, they were gone.

On June 15th, three days after joining our family and putting up an intense fight, Morgan received her baby Angel wings. I remember getting the call in the middle of the night. I was still in the hospital after delivering my girls via an emergency C-section. The nurse on the other end of the phone said, "We've given her the highest amount of oxygen we can, and she is not responding. Her ventilator is at the highest setting, which is unhealthy for her and hard on her underdeveloped lungs. We think you should come down." As my husband and I walked down to the NICU, I called my family, he called his family and we prepared to say goodbye to our daughter. The mood in the NICU was sad, an indescribable feeling I will never forget. Morgan's doctors and nurses looked like they had run a marathon. I could tell they had been working on baby girl and worked like hell to keep her alive. They had only been keeping her on the ventilator until we arrived. When we arrived, many words were said and many questions were asked. The only thing I remember from that conversation was that Morgan would not survive through the night. It was time to say goodbye. The nurse offered to dress Morgan in all white instead of the diaper and onesie she was wearing. She pulled out this beautiful white bonnet and a beautiful white gown; she looked like an Angel. It was time, Morgan was taken out of the incubator, and the ventilator was removed. Morgan was placed in my arms, and I remember looking into her eyes to let her know it was ok to rest now. She had already changed my life forever. My heart shattered into what felt like a million pieces at that moment. Morgan took four little breaths, her eyes closed, and she was gone. And just like that, I became a mom to a deceased infant child. This was not a miscarriage like the babies before; the daughter I birthed died in my arms.

Life can be funny or cruel depending on how you view it. You make elaborate plans, envision how perfect things will be, and then somewhere along the journey, those plans change. One thing I know for sure, nothing in this life prepares you for losing a child. Nothing prepares you for losing two children.

After losing Morgan, although sad, we didn't have time to let the grief of losing one child set in. Ryan was still fighting and, as a mom, my only goal at that moment was to put all my energy into ensuring Ryan survived. I asked all the questions, read the books, and asked about skin-to-skin contact, and in the end, none of it mattered. On July 2nd, we received another call. As we drove to the hospital at 2:30 am, the tears that had streamed down my face so often - every day to be honest - already began to flow again. I'd already lost one daughter. Although my faith was shattered and I was angry with God, I prayed that I would not lose another child. As we took the long walk through the hospital to the

NICU, the smell of sadness took over my nose. I can still smell the halls of the empty hospital even though I have not stepped foot in it since July 2, 2015. As we walked into Ryan's room, the doctors and nurses were working on her. However, today was different; her room was bright and jumping; it was typically dark or dimly lit. All of the lights were on, the machines were beeping and people were running back and forth. There was an airlift team ready to take my baby to another hospital. Unfortunately, we would later find out that the medical staff could not stabilize her, so the team was unable to move her. As the doctors and nurses moved around, I grabbed my baby girl's tiny hand and placed my finger in her hand. As her tiny fingers wrapped around my pointer finger, the bells and alarms stopped. I kissed her forehead. Ryan took a few breaths, and then she was gone. I watched my 2nd daughter take her last breath. I have never experienced something so beautiful and painfully earth-shattering simultaneously to this day. It's a feeling of sadness that has never left me and will stop me in my tracks at any moment.

From the moment I met Ryan and Morgan and was able to hold my daughters, I remember feeling incredibly blessed, even through all the fear and sadness that comes with life in the NICU. I remember when my daughters passed, how they looked at me with the most beautiful eyes as they each took their last breaths, and in both moments, I prayed that God would stop their suffering. When you love someone unconditionally, it's the best kind of love, but it's also about what you give, not what you receive. I fully understand why people say children are the heartbeat outside their bodies. I felt this way about Ryan and Morgan, I felt it for the babies we miscarried, and I feel it now for our four-year-old son.

I will never forget their adorable little faces and those tiny hands and feet! While that experience was filled with sadness, there were also many days of happiness. My faith has slowly been restored, and I continually thank God each day for our little blessings. We will never forget how much joy they brought to our lives and the lives of family and friends who were fortunate enough to have met them. Although they were only with us for a short period, their lives mattered, and they will forever live in our hearts, and we will love them forever. We will never forget Ryan and Morgan, affectionately named the "Tinymights."

It's been seven years since we had to say goodbye to our daughters, and in those seven years, we have experienced several failed IUIs, IVF cycles and several miscarriages. We've also experienced so much joy from the birth of our rainbow baby, who turned four years old this year. I was also able to start an event planning business in Ryan and Morgan's memory. *RyanMorgan Events* has hosted retreats for moms who have lost or are living with infertility. I've also coached families through several rounds of IVF. I am always willing to share my story and support women who have to travel this lonely road. It brings me so much joy to do what friends and family did and continue to do for me.

Someone once said that loving and grieving one baby while loving another is the ultimate balancing act as a parent, and I couldn't agree with this statement more. I love my son with every fiber of my being, but it still does not stop the emptiness I feel from losing two living children. I have been pregnant five times, and I have one surviving child. Losing children taught me that nothing in life is guaranteed, but my son and a good therapist remind me daily that anything is possible. I hold on to THAT joy daily!

I encourage you to find your joy if you are part of this "club" and hold on to it. Bottle it up for the rough days on this journey. You will need them! This journey is full of peaks and valleys, highs and lows. I've learned that the ups and downs do not last forever and that mindfully being grateful for each moment of my journey has brought me so much joy. As painful as it has been, I am thankful for it all and continue to speak joy over my life, family and son. It's been good for my soul.

Courtney Shorter, a native Washingtonian, currently resides in PG County with her husband, son and fur baby. Obsessed with planning events and parties, and fascinated by all the details in dressing up, dancing, the music, lights, the food, and the glamour, she is the owner and Chief Event Officer of RyanMorgan Events. Named after her twin angel babies, Ryan and Morgan, her company is built on a bedrock of love, a passion for what's possible and a commitment to be an unstoppable force for good! Much like a stylist she helps her clients find the best garments to showcase the greatest versions of who they are, "I help my clients throw the best party or event to exhibit the very best of what they have to offer."

As a way to honor her babies after many years of event planning and heartbreak, RyanMorgan Events recently extended their business offerings to empower women who have experienced infant loss, miscarriages and/or women who are living with infertility. Soul Free Mamas was created as a powerful space for women that crave to be heard and supported along this lonely journey.

The Courage of Life through Infertility

by Tiffany Thompson

After three years of marriage, my family reminded me that I had not started building my own family. Time flies when you are a newly wedded couple and having fun.

After completing my college education, I started a new career which sometimes kept me out late. Merging the thought of returning home to prepare dinner for two and the concern of having children was quite overwhelming, but I had to be strong and think positive. However, being strong became somewhat difficult during this journey.

I knew I had Polycystic Ovarian Syndrome (PCOS) but was oblivious to the future infertility journey. I was unprepared for anything besides the usual way of getting pregnant to complete my family. To think that it was more than a year of intentionally trying to produce babies for those efforts to seem futile. Officially, this period marked the beginning of the bothersome journey.

The doctor, ultrasound technician and blood lab technicians schooled me through PCOS education to begin my promising future of being a mother.

While going through an infertility journey, your conscience reminds you that your best moment is yet to come. My loveliest moment was when I was self-motivated - the fact that I was determined not to throw in the towel leaves me in awe.

Although it took a while to decide never to give up my dream of being a mother, I was determined amidst my pains that I would carry babies.

Metal was the smell I encountered when I was being wheeled down to the operating room numerous times to have yet another dilation and curettage (D&C) procedure. The metal smell was significant as it reminded me for the time I wanted to give up.

When I smell metal today, my mind flashes back to the physical and mental pain of what I said and how it had become normal for me. My brain has normalized the pains like it was something trivial. I was on the second D&C procedure in two days and the second miscarriage of twin babies. Losing a pregnancy puts one's mental health in a tight corner.

Emotionally, I couldn't bear the pain my body was enduring and the mental disruptions I was going through. I could not reason that some of this was beyond my control. My husband, Jesse, was doing all he could to mentally and physically be there for me while trying to compose himself and deal with his own heartache.

After HCG injections, I developed fluid accumulation within my uterine cavity. I was going through the IVF process and was taking HCG injections to stimulate the development of eggs in my ovaries. The swelling and fluid accumulation in my abdomen caused my ovaries to swell and become painful. Thinking of all the visits to the doctor, I had to get liters of fluid drained from my stomach. My mind became overwhelmed with negative thoughts

The severity of this process felt like intentional physical torture. It was a traumatic moment in the doctor's office. I fidgeted as I watched the doctor drain off as much fluid as possible. Laying on the bed, all I could think of was the horror of not being able to have children after all that I have been through.

Drifting off into my feelings, I pictured my future without children. The miscarriages were beyond my control. The doctor would always say the loss is no one's fault. Sometimes, it happens whether you do things right or do them the other way. It took a while for me to overcome and comprehend what the doctor told me.

The mental frustration was not allowing me to focus on the bigger picture. At that moment, I thought of giving up on my dream of becoming a mother. After suffering consecutive miscarriages, we decided to step back and take a break. My husband and I had to recharge and gain control of our lives mentally. We had to realize that it would happen when the time was right. When God said the time is right.

During this journey, you will assume every minute to be the worst moment. I had gotten the news once again that I was pregnant. Blood levels had increased weekly and I felt all the symptoms of being pregnant. Again, we became excited, but immediately became uncomfortable while checking out a new house with my husband and the realtor. The thought of having a new house and being pregnant should have been one of the happiest moments of my life. But that memory took a slight turn.

I went to the bathroom at the potential home and looked in the mirror. Before I encountered the next step, I had to pray. I had to engage God at the moment. The feeling in my heart made me know that the unexpected was about to happen, and it would not be appealing. I looked down at my leg, and I was hemorrhaging.

Immediately, I knew it was time to schedule an appointment to have yet another dilation and curettage. This period was bad because every woman knows hemorrhaging equals no baby. I cried and prayed all night. Finally, I garnered enough courage to call the emergency number.

While waiting for the doctor to call back, I tried to prepare myself mentally for the worst that loomed ahead. The doctor called back and immediately scheduled for me to come the next day to talk about options and the process for me to get rid of the pregnancy. My emotions were numb.

During the night, all I could do was brood how optimistic I was about carrying this baby to full term (successful pregnancy), but it seemed like things would turn out bad.

My regular doctor called to tell me to wait another week. Although I am in the know that "PCOS women may sometimes ovulate a week later, and the hemorrhaging could be harmless", I was hesitant. The tears, the constant tremble, the prayers and the faith were dominant during my infertility journey. God was all that I could hold onto for a better composure.

I listened and followed through with my doctor's advice. After waiting a week and still hemorrhaging, I made a visit of fate to the lab. The ultrasound room was dark, cold and quiet. I went in for an ultrasound, and to our surprise, we saw her. My rainbow baby, her heartbeat.

After learning of PCOS and going through a couple of miscarriages, hearing my rainbow baby cry while on the operating table was the favorite moment of my journey. While in the operating room, I took note of the instructions for each step. After a short while, the doctor notified me that it was time. I was fascinated that the baby would be out at any moment. I never felt pressure or contractions and did not hear my baby cry.

My heart started palpitating almost immediately. My husband saw the tears running down my cheeks and quickly notified the medical staff that I was worried because I did not hear my baby cry. All the pain I felt during my infertility journey came back to me; having to deal with the horrible smell of metal in the operating room, enduring the sad news of not carrying a viable pregnancy, the excruciating cramps that accompany hemorrhaging, the daily visit to the hospital, HCG injections, the draining of fluid and the ultrasounds of cysts all played back in my memory when my husband confirmed my baby was delivered but not crying.

A couple of minutes later, my rainbow baby finally cried, and the tears of pain turned into tears of joy. The pains of the prior unsuccessful pregnancies disappeared into thin air. Eventually, I birthed a baby - that I heard crying and was confirmed to look healthy. It was a euphoric moment of surprise and happiness. After having 15 hours of labor, pushing and then an emergency c-section due to the cord wrapped around my baby's neck, I had already expected the worst. But still, fortunately, the outcome became the best moment of my infertility journey.

Looking into my daughter's eyes for the first time was a dream come true. It was like time stood still for a moment. We gazed at each other like, "hey, I know you. I heard your voice all the time, and I finally got to see your face and hold you." We felt the connection instantly, and at that moment, I knew that all the trials and struggles to get to this point were all worth it. I would not trade this moment for anything. Now, we are enjoying the fruits of our labor, well, my labor.

Although my husband did not experience labor pain, he did experience weight gain and morning sickness. So together we experienced a difficult pregnancy with a successful outcome. However, we were always grateful to God for the journey. It was a bumpy ride, but with prayers and belief, we achieved our goal of becoming parents.

If I were to describe my journey in five sentences, I'd love to note that it was a mixture of emotions. It was sometimes overwhelming. At one point, it became a learning process. It unveiled our determination, motivation and the feeling that we can conquer whatever comes our way.

The journey heightened the bond between myself and my husband.

My husband and I went through depression, ups and downs, fear and the thought of giving up. Not one day had gone by that we did not speak of having a family. I was never alone; he followed through with all decisions and complied with everything the doctor ordered.

He did not go through the pain physically, but he mentally coped and held onto his feelings separate from mine.

Dealing with the mental effect of multiple miscarriages causes moments of disbelief, and you start to question why. Then the depression starts to kick in because all you can think about are the what-ifs. Trying to be present for your spouse to keep them motivated because you know that they are in pain also. It is painful to see the one you love hurting, but you must keep holding on to your faith and let God take the lead.

It took a while to want to talk about what I was feeling without wet stuff spilling out of my eyes. Times when nothing made me happy and I did not want to leave my room, moments that I did not want to smile, my husband was there every step of the way. It would have been harder bearing those awful experiences alone.

My rainbow baby has filled the vacuum I had in my heart. As I look back and remember all we had been through to conceive a baby, I would not change any of the factors.

My faith in God prepared and molded me to be the best parent I can be. I was angry. No one understood what I was going through. I had no one to lean on and cry out my sorrows. I was cranky most of the time, and I transferred aggression to my husband who was also battling depression.

It was hard to deal with my emotions and try to be there for him. Casting my mind back to my journey, I do not expect others to feel sorry for us or mention good intentions that may not have happened, but to help people with similar challenges cope with the process.

Not that our trials and tribulation are more significant than any other couple or family, just that we have been through our years of tested faith.

Many family and friends did not know the details of the infertility journey, some were just aware of the miscarriages. However, they had words of comfort and wisdom which held a special place in our hearts. They would say things like “keep your faith” and “do not give up. It will happen in time.” They would also offer to share their experiences with having gone through miscarriages.

God was working on it. He was working on a masterpiece that represents us. But, of course, God was right, as we all know He does not make mistakes. The colors were perfect and the images were immaculate. The tenderness of the cheek was a delight on its own. The softness of the melanin tone skin was an ideal mixture of mom and dad. The artist knew our struggles and decided that the work of art had to be perfect for us. So, we were compensated a million folds for our trouble. She was indeed the coolness of our eyes.

Bonding with our baby was what we wanted so badly.

My family not knowing the struggles that we went through during infertility is the reason for my story. It's hard talking to families who have never experienced infertility. But, knowing that I hid it from my loved ones made me think that others who face similar challenges need to hear my story to assure them that they are not alone.

I had a swell time meeting my daughter for the first time. It felt so surreal wrapping her in my arms.

Looking into her eyes as I lay on the operating table is a moment I will never forget. Frequent phone calls, doctor visits, stress, heartache, tears, depression and years of pain were all that I endured during my journey.

Never would I have thought that this story of mine would be worth telling—my dark moments of thinking that there was no way over the hump. My rainbow baby has brought my family much joy and happiness. We do not cease to celebrate the gift given to us and the journey that brought my family closer.

Many families are trying to conceive and it seems like an uphill battle; the obstacles are constantly getting in the way, making you want to throw in the towel. Please keep striving and praying, and your dream of becoming a parent will come true.

I have thought about giving up. After failed pregnancies, infertility injections, and fluid accumulation from the IVF process, I felt that my body could no longer take it. The trauma was unbearable. The depression and the time were painful. I had to take a moment and think, "is it worth it?" I had put my life on hold for years to try and complete my family.

We pushed through. We were reminiscing about all miscarriages, surgeries, high-risk pregnancies and the scary delivery. I have decided that my rainbow baby was all worth it. She completes our family.

Love letter to Heaven Briann Thompson (Rainbow baby): One night in a dream, God came with words of wisdom. He spoke with such conviction that you were meant to be our dream that will one day come true. Therefore, we named you Heaven. Though we waited for a while, we are glad you arrived at that time. You were our little gift from God. Our love for you is unconditional and you are so amazing. You fill our hearts with joy and we thank God daily for the journey of infertility. You were worth it. You did not know it before, but as you read this love letter, you will see that you're our most precious blessing from God.

Tiffany Ann-Griffin Thompson is a wife, mother, daughter, aunt, and sister that aspires to stay consistent with efforts to be better for herself, family and her community. She founded her own healthcare services business in which she provides Revenue Cycle Management services for Healthcare services. She is the founder of Maximal Business Healthcare Service. She is originally from Richmond, Virginia, but her work and professional obligations have led to her to travel to meet the needs of her chosen communities. Tiffany is an active, vibrant and curious individual with a charming and enigmatic personality that helps her captivate, inspire, and influence others. She is always very enthusiastic about leveraging her expertise to run her business and reach her goals effectively. With almost two decades of experience in the healthcare sector and a degree in Healthcare Administration, she ensures she gets the job done in the right way and is very successful in her career. Through her work in the field, Tiffany has gained the first-hand experience necessary for success in senior management roles and has also worked with many NGOs to further her cause.

Tiffany is a leader and takes responsibility for any assignment and works effectively with people from different backgrounds and organizations. She has also achieved numerous milestones and earned a string of recognitions and accolades for her distinguished services in the Healthcare field. Tiffany enjoys spending time with her family, traveling and catching up on a good read. Tiffany's next phase in her life is to help families overcome the journey of infertility.

2 Rainbows for 2 Storms

by Terika Williams

I dedicate this work to my unborn babies. Although I did not get a chance to meet you, you have made a profound impact on my life and for that I am forever grateful. To my amazing daughters, thank you for bringing so much love and joy into my life. I hope that my telling of this story encourages you to continue to be brave, walk in your brilliance, and do the scary things in life. To my wonderful husband, none of this would be possible without you. Thank you for being the yin to my yang, for being my rock, and for always encouraging and pushing me. You helped me to endure all of life's difficult moments and for that I love you beyond measure.

I pray that this submission helps someone who is experiencing or has experienced a miscarriage. I hope my words provide some relief in knowing that you are not alone, and that you will make it through this difficult time. I hope you understand that this unfortunate occurrence is not your fault and that countless other women share in your experience and your pain while also knowing that there can be joy on the other side. I hope this book helps us to be more willing to have these conversations so that women no longer feel like they have to suffer in silence. And most importantly, I encourage you to keep going when you are in the midst of a storm because there is a reward on the other side.

Like with many of the other things in my life, this opportunity just seemed to find me. My co-author and good girlfriend brought the opportunity to my attention and, initially, I did not think much of it. I did not think that my story was important enough to share because there are so many other women who have had experiences far greater than mine. A while later, she sent me the recording of the initial meeting and I probably would have swept the thought under the rug again had I not just had my quarterly energy reading. In the reading, I was informed that I needed to "share my story outside of my immediate circle." This message came to me at exactly the right time and made me think that I could actually do this. I must also mention that in my very first energy reading, I was informed that I would write a book about children. As I am not a writer and not involved with children outside of my own and my family, I disregarded this information as well because yeah right, that's not me at all. But here we are almost two years later and the opportunity has presented itself. It has come nearly full circle. And while I still do not completely feel like my story is as significant as some other's I will not let this chance pass me by. Here is my story.

As the mother of two beautiful daughters, I am frequently asked "are you guys going to try for a boy?" (I do not understand why so many people feel comfortable asking these types of questions, but they do). The answer is always "no" but, depending on who asked, they may get a little more detail. If the person is close to me, I may explain that I have been pregnant four times, two ending in miscarriage and two resulting in our beautiful rainbow babies. Additionally, I will add that I am terrified of having twins, my mother is a twin and with age and number of pregnancies, my chances of having twins has increased. What I typically do not say is that I believe deep in my heart that my two miscarriages were my boys and I carry them with me.

Finding out we were pregnant the first time was very exciting! It was Thanksgiving (how appropriate). My husband and I took the pregnancy test that morning and I proceeded to make my first peach cobbler for the family dinner; now it is the dish that is expected of me at every holiday meal. As it was my first time making the dessert, I was not aware that I needed to drain some of the juice from the peaches and when I went to remove it from the oven the hot juice rolled down my left arm and burned me. But we had just received the best news of our married life so we could not let that ruin our day, right? Right! My husband helped me wrap it up and we went to dinner later and shared our news during the famous black family tradition of going around the table and saying what you are thankful for. Everyone was so happy for us because they had been asking since we got married when we were going to start trying (there goes those questions again). Never did it cross my mind that we would have a miscarriage. Looking back, I understand now that you can never take a pregnancy for granted but back then I was young and naive. Days later I started to spot. I still wasn't worried because a miscarriage was not on my radar. We were young and healthy and more importantly, no one EVER talked about miscarriages. I really wish the women I knew would have felt more comfortable sharing those parts of their story with us. I wish it wasn't such a silent burden to bear. When the bleeding did not stop, my doctor told us to go to the emergency room and it was confirmed that we indeed had a miscarriage. I also had my burn looked at (which I definitely should have done earlier) and treated. To this day, I have a scar on my left arm that looks like a uterus. To me, it reminds me of that first pregnancy. Because we announced so early that we were pregnant, we had to deal with well-meaning people asking about the progress after the miscarriage. That most certainly was a secondary trauma that I did not expect. Every time someone else asked when the baby was due or how the pregnancy was coming along, it felt like reliving the loss over again. Needless to say, we learned our lesson and did not tell many people about the other pregnancies until after it felt safer to do so.

After waiting the suggested three months for my body to heal, we got pregnant with our first rainbow baby. While I loved being pregnant, every time I was, the joy of it all was overshadowed by the fear of losing the baby. At every sonogram and every appointment, there is a hint of fear. We made it to full-term where she made us wait an additional two days to meet her. She was due on a Friday. The doctor sent us to the hospital because my blood pressure was up but after a few hours they sent us home. The next day, we went back because my contractions were coming every five minutes. Still, they sent us back home. Sunday morning, my father called and asked "you aren't ready to have that baby yet?" I told him apparently she wasn't ready. A little while later, my water broke and finally the hospital couldn't turn us away. I labored for hours but did not dilate, the doctor came in and said I could have a C-section then or wait until the morning. I was beyond ready so C-section it was. Once she was finally here and we could hold her I could finally breathe. I felt like whatever I did wrong or whatever was not right in my body the first time had corrected itself. I felt less of a failure. A couple of years later, we were ready to try again. Fortunately, we are a very fertile couple and getting pregnant has been fairly easy for us. So here we are, pregnancy number three and this one lasted longer than number one but not long enough for us to announce. I was speaking with my aunt the other day and she stated that she did not even know about this pregnancy. We went for a sonogram appointment and I could see on the technician's face that something was wrong. She said "the baby is measuring smaller than it should." The doctor later confirmed what I expected: we had another miscarriage. This time there was no physical scar to accompany the loss but we had to schedule a D&C. I cannot describe how utterly heartbreaking it is to drive to the hospital to have them remove a lifeless baby from your womb. That is a different kind of trauma. This time, there were fewer questions as only a handful of people knew.

Together, we made it through another loss and decided to try again and we had our second rainbow baby. This pregnancy too was filled with fear. She was planned as I did not want to be pregnant in the summer again, nor did I want to deal with issues we had with our eldest regarding her late birthday and the start of the school year. She was conceived in Las Vegas and we have an adorable picture of her in a onesie that says "I'm what happened in Vegas." One day on the way to training for work, I slipped and fell on a piece of ice at the Metro station. On top of all the other fears I had about losing babies, I beat myself up for this. How could I be so careless? If anything happened to this baby I would have no doubt it would totally have been my fault. Her birth was a scheduled C-section on March 9th at 7 am so that was my standard answer when asked when she was due. I had the option of trying to have her naturally if she came before our appointed time, but just like her older sister she would not budge. I probably should have known she would give me a run for my money after she refused my first request of her: to allow me to have her vaginally. Because her birth was scheduled I did not have many contractions (I am in NO way complaining about that) but I really did want to try to have her vaginally. Having two C-sections is another thing I grappled with, that made me feel like I did not truly experience the birthing process. It's crazy how many expectations are placed upon expectant mothers, both internally and externally.

I have always believed that everything happens for a reason and when it is supposed to. So while I do not physically have any sons, I do believe with my entire heart that I have carried two boys in my body, no matter how short a period of time. I will forever carry them in my heart. My two rainbow babies are the most precious, loving, smart girls I know and I am extremely grateful for them.

Terika Williams was born and raised in Prince George's County, Maryland where she currently resides with her husband, two daughters and dog. She is a graduate of the University of Maryland, Baltimore County where she graduated with a degree in Psychology and a minor in Social Work. She currently works as a Community Supervision Officer. Prior to this position, she worked with autistic children in a position that provided her with great satisfaction. She has always had a passion for helping others and hopes her addition to this book does just that.

Terika is a wife, mother, daughter, sister, aunt and friend. She enjoys spending time with her family and friends. The activity does not matter, it can be as simple as relaxing at home or at someone else's home or as extravagant as traveling to different countries. Being with those she loves simply feeds her soul. She also loves to read!

She has been described as a dependable person who is very caring. If you need someone to be there for you in your time of need or to provide a listening ear, she's your person. Although being supportive is a significant part of her DNA, actually being involved in writing this book is completely out of her comfort zone and she hopes that the readers enjoy her contribution.

CONCLUSION

More than five million people in the United States experience some type of infertility, miscarriage or infant loss. Although this type of trauma is widely acknowledged as something that affects millions of families, many families still feel ashamed, hopeless, and isolated.

Studies have shown that infertile couples experience significant anxiety and emotional distress.

A diagnosis of infertility can be emotionally and physically challenging - leading to depression and isolation. Even after successfully conceiving, the loss of a baby during pregnancy remains a sad reality for many families. According to the CDC, 24,000 stillbirths were reported in the United States in 2017. The same study found that Black mothers were more than twice as likely to experience stillbirth compared to Hispanic and white mothers.

A study from Seminars in Fetal & Neonatal Medicine contends that families struggle to cope with the immediate and long-lasting effects of a baby's death which can last for years and sometimes decades. We tend to regard sacrifice, loss, strength, and vulnerability as the hallmarks of parenthood.

Resilience Rising is an intimate compilation of stories by families living with infertility who have experienced pregnancy and infant loss and are choosing to live, be Resilient, and share their experience while celebrating moments of joy through this process. We hope that this book empowers you or someone you love to do the same.

Made in the USA
Middletown, DE
06 October 2022

11851871R10086